BEJI

MW01265632

Awakening the Light Within

Gia Govinda Marie

Blessings & Light
Gia

A Collection of Powerful
Affirmations & Writings
To Assist Humanity's Awakening
Into the Golden Age of Light

Llumina
Press

ISBN: 978-1-60594-279-7

Printed in the United States of America by Llumina Press

Library of Congress Control Number: 2009902482

May this book assist you in your soul's Conscious Awakening Process, igniting and integrating the codes deep within your core, preparing you for humanity's ascension process as you move into the Golden Age of Light, co-creating beautifully with Spirit.

Love, light & radiance to you on your most sacred journey home.

DEDICATION

To my beautiful mom, Jena Brayton Hausknecht, who has ALWAYS believed in me, with unwavering faith, and who never questioned the steps on my journey.

ACKNOWLEDGMENTS

Special thanks to Divine Spirit, the loving Angels, Guides, Ascended Masters, and Teachers that have graced me with their presence through the years.

Thank you also "Beings of Light" and Nature Spirits for your gentle, but enthusiastic guidance every step of the way. To my beautiful daughter, Camille, who is my inspiration and hero. To my spiritual family and friends… each and every one of you knows who you are, as you have helped me weave the colorful tapestry of my life on this plane.

Special acknowledgment to my beloved friend, Ann, who crossed over during the creation of this book, who continues to work with her team of Angels on the other side and shower us with blessings. To Elfie, Katy, and Alisa for your unending encouragement and support. You are shining lights in my life.

And finally, to my "inner child" who incessantly reached out to me until she was heard, as we continue our journey hand-in-hand.

~ I am full of gratitude and love for you all ~

INTRODUCTION

Our existence on the earth plane is a spiritual quest. Each of us here has a soul's mission we are to awaken to and fulfill. We are in the midst of a long-awaited shift on the planet, ushering humanity into the new Age of Light, and although we are in the human form, we are Spiritual Beings awakening to the full potential of who we are and what gifts we are to share with the world.

The information in this book is nothing new. It is ancient wisdom passed down through the ages by the Ascended Masters and other Celestial Beings who have chosen to assist humanity on the earth plane to awaken and remind the masses of who they truly are and what they are here to do.

It is my sincere hope and desire that each of you reading these words fully resonates with the beauty of your soul as you embark on your journey of self-discovery.

Because a portion of this book is channeled information, it has not been altered, but intentionally preserved in its original format of transmission to keep the messages clear and authentic.

Blessings & Gratitude,
Gia

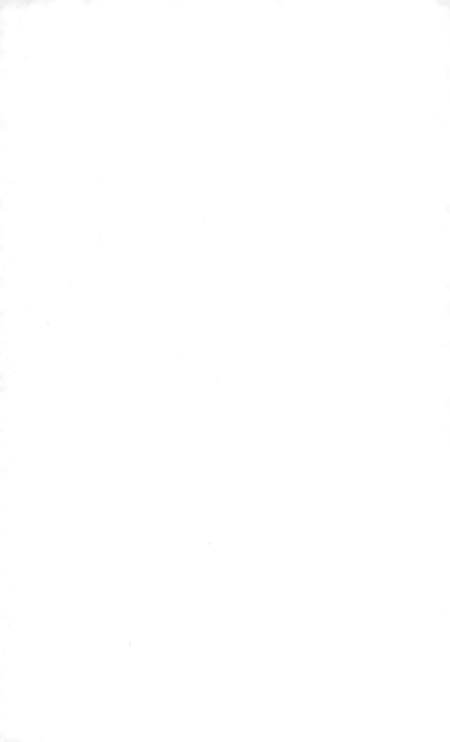

Throughout these writings are italicized excerpts provided by the "Beings of Light", who are Divine Beings, Angels, Ascended Masters, and other beautiful Cosmic Guides who have assisted me in the knowledge shared heretofore.

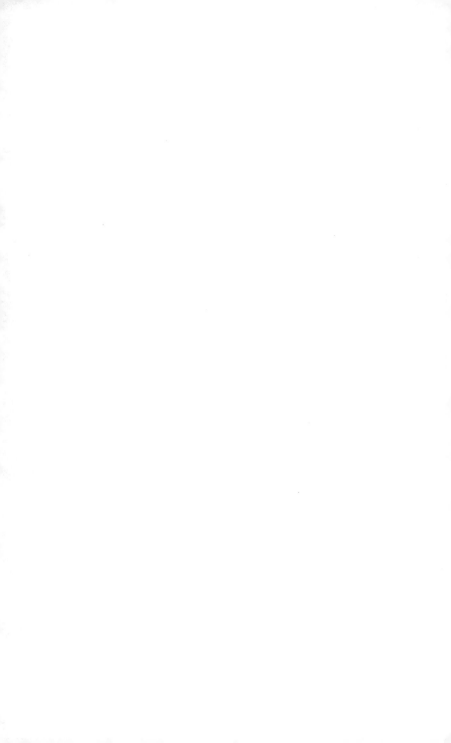

PART 1

As humanity continues to increase its vibrational frequency on the earth plane, we have come to a universal pivotal point, where it is more vital than ever before to truly *realize* the effect of not only our spoken words, but our thought forms as well. The Ascended Masters and other Celestial Beings have brought us this powerful knowledge and information throughout the years, and we have reached a critical point in our evolution to embrace these teachings and transform our lives. May these affirmations and writings guide and assist you on your soul's journey home and in your Conscious Awakening process.

OM NAMAHA SHIVAYA

Greetings Dear Ones,

We come to you from the ethers of Shamballa at the Temple of Enlightened Ones. May these words be embraced by your hearts and may your inner lights blaze brightly, radiating love, peace, and healing energy to the world.

We Are,
The Beings of Light

PART 2

As I have traveled my spiritual path, I've come to realize that it is most valuable to create and utilize I AM affirmations, as they immediately connect one with the Christ Consciousness field, zooming the intention out into the universe at an incredibly vast speed. As always, it is good practice to instill affirmations into your mind and consciousness that do <u>not</u> contain no, not, don't, etc., as the subconscious does not translate and assimilate the negative rhythm of these words.

These affirmations will shift your vibrational frequency almost instantaneously. Set aside some quiet space every morning after you arise, visualize your day unfolding in a magical way, and speak your affirmations. Soon, you will begin to see miraculous changes occurring in your life.

Fine tune and create your own affirmations, repeating each one three times before going on to the next.

You may also chant or sing your affirmations, for the beauty of the emotional force assists the deep intention of your decrees and is delightful to the Beings in the Spiritual and Angelic Kingdoms.

THE "CANCEL" EFFECT:

There are times, of course, when we say things that may not be of our highest intent. After all, we are in the human body and this is the learning plane. . . This is where the "CANCEL" effect comes into play. . . It's quite simple and actually recalibrates our energy field when applied. And, in these times when we are consciously recoding, reconnecting, and reactivating our energetic matrixes, it is imperative to keep our cells regenerated and clear of negative memory.

For example, when you find yourself speaking a fearful or negative statement, whether it's about yourself or someone else, immediately state the word "CANCEL!" (i.e., "I can't do anything right!" CANCEL!). And, to transform the statement at an even deeper level, I would invite you to replace that initial thought or statement with a positive one, like, "I AM divinely guided in every area of my life and am standing in my empowerment now!" Follow this practice and watch your life change in glorious ways.

The "Cancel" effect is the soft lotus flower that patiently waits beneath us when we stumble, beautifully placing us back on our mark to continue our movement forward on our path.

PART 3

The affirmations in this book are intended to be fully absorbed, integrating and assimilating divine KNOWINGNESS deep within your soul, thus assisting you in your full Conscious Awakening Process.

I AM one with God

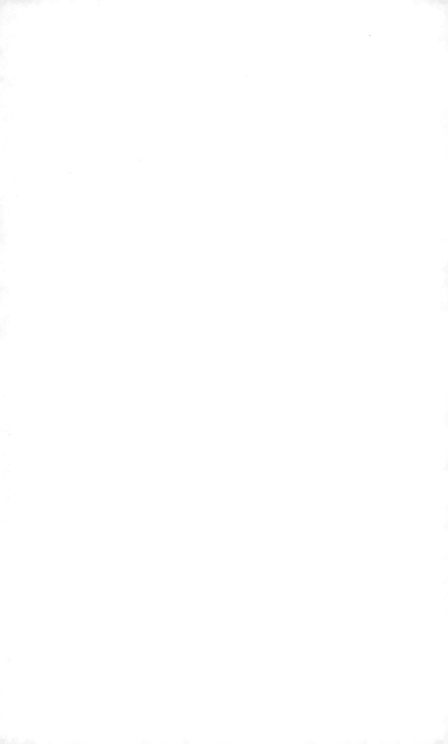

I AM one with my Higher Self

My soul and my personality
are in perfect alignment!

Greetings Dear Ones,

We come to you on this day, each and every one of you reading these words, to awaken within you a deeper clarity and understanding of the Divine Word and Cosmic Alignment that is preparing to take place on your most recent place of origin, Planet Earth. Those of you who have sought out these words are here to play a very important role in the Ascension plan, and we honor you for answering the call, for it is only those courageously soaring into their spiritual missions that are needed NOW!

Many of you are questioning events that are going on in your lives at this time, and may be wondering about the significance and necessity of these happenings. What we would like to tell you at this time, Dear Ones, is that these perceived challenges or obstacles are actually igniting and fueling you for the transformative Ascension process. For if everything was flowing along smoothly in your incarnations, why would you even **think** *to explore the higher dimensional meaning of Light. It is through challenge and perceived darkness that light can emerge. The beauty of the Awakening Soul can be compared to the unrecognizable lotus bud that is deeply submerged beneath the murkiest of mud and mire. When suddenly, upon divine timing, the tender, vulnerable bud gloriously emerges to the surface, and upon embracing the bright light, opens up and blossoms into the most beautiful wonder of nature.*

The bud of awakening has opened in each and every one of you reading these words and it is now time to REMEMBER WHO YOU ARE at your deepest core level. We love you dearly and shall guide you on your journey always.

We Are,
The Beings of Light

I AM fulfilling my Spiritual Mission now!

I AM recalibrating and realigning
my energy system into my highest
Spiritual Essence & Divine Blueprint now!

I AM fully connected & beautifully aligned
with the three-fold flame within my heart

*Call out Dear Ones, for you
cannot be answered, if you are not heard . . .
The Messengers of Light await patiently and hold the
field for the murmur of your intentions, as you co-create
with Spirit in preparation for your entrance into the
Golden Age of Light . . .*

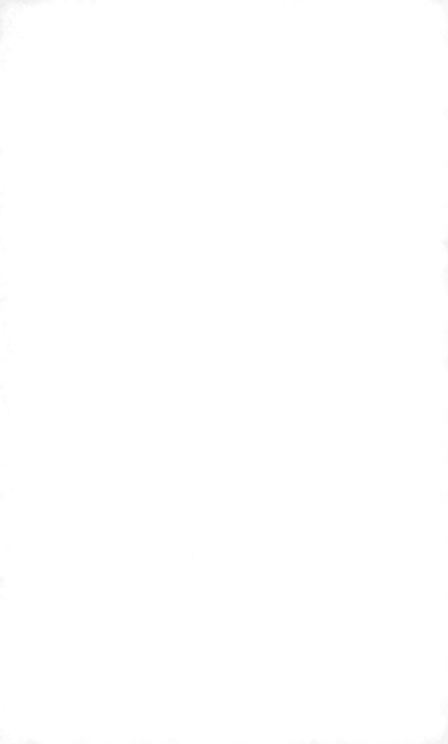

I AM vibrating in my highest
frequency and truth now!

I AM speaking with the "Voice of My Heart"
in each and every moment!

I AM communicating clearly
with all of my enlightened Angels,
Guides, Ascended Masters & Teachers!

I AM radiating love & harmony
to ALL humanity now!

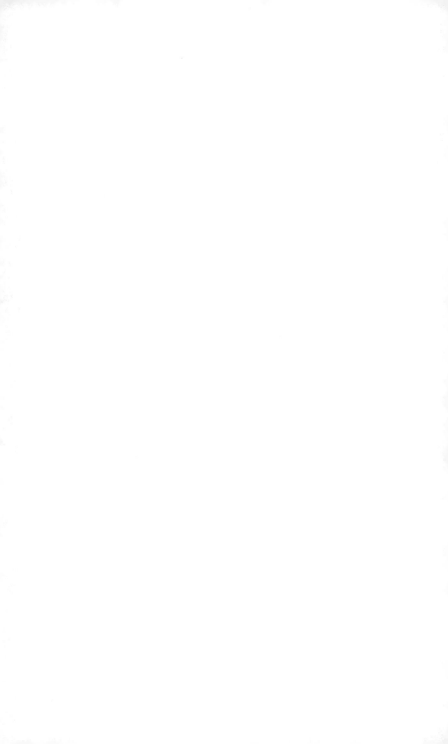

Greetings Dear Ones,

We come to you on wings of the dove, ushering in love, peace, and joy to you on this day. We have been hearing in multitude, questions encircling your consciousness and the urgency upon which the answers are sought. We bless you for your enthusiasm in unlocking the Secret Chamber of your hearts, for within this mystical treasure box sleeps the destiny of your soul. Many of you are questioning your incarnations at this time. Why am I here? What IS it that I am here to do? We applaud you, for this Dear Ones, is the first step of your journey home. Ask and you shall receive. Have faith, Dear Ones, unwavering faith, that your divine destiny is unfolding at this very moment in perfect and profound order.

Let me ask you this question, Children of Light, what method of service to humanity would make your heart sing? If you could select anything in the world that brings you joy, and provides assistance and divine service to your brothers and sisters, what would that be? Know and believe that you can accomplish this. So many times in human incarnations, earthlings LIMIT themselves with self-doubt and negative thought forms, sabotaging the very essence of who they are. It is now time to release the illusional chains that bind your field, that hold you back from stepping into your true divine nature, and share your gifts with the world. Each soul here has a specific mission to fulfill, but most do not awaken to the Light of Consciousness. We salute you on your journey and prepare your path of gold ahead.

Blessings & Peace.

We Are,
The Beings of Light

I AM receiving my spiritual directives
to fulfill my soul's purpose now!

I AM fully stepping into my life's work,
and doing what I AM here to do!

I AM glowing in inner illumination!

Greetings Dear Ones,

At this time of great acceleration of Christ Consciousness on the planet, it is necessary for the Alliance of Light Workers to step into full attention as we bring forth these ancient teachings into your energy fields. As you breathe in this Golden Liquid Light, you cleanse and reprogram any negative memories of long ago and of many incarnations, saturating every cell of your bodies with love, light, and the divine frequency of Spirit . . .

We Are,
The Beings of Light

I AM a fully awakened,
multidimensional, conscious Spiritual Being!

I AM communicating clearly
with my Higher Self in each and every moment!

I AM one with
Divine Clarity & Pure Understanding!

I AM living my truth
and standing in my empowerment now!

Greetings & Blessings, Dear Ones,

The technographics of the Spiritual Energy Field resembles a magnificent jewel with many intricate facets that glisten and sparkle at every angle. Be Who You Are Dear Ones. It is time to step into the Beauty of Who You Are and create your true destiny on the earth plane. Let go of any fear or doubt. Trust, KNOW, and BELIEVE that you are a magnificent Being, shimmering in the Light of Spirit and that ALL is possible. . .

Blessings,
The Beings of Light

I AM releasing and clearing any
fear & negativity from ALL levels of my Beingness and
my cellular memory forevermore!

I AM infused with good nature
and I AM sharing this energy with the world now!

I AM in superb balance
physically, emotionally, mentally & spiritually

I AM living in the energy
of love, purity & happiness now!

Dear Ones,

We gather on this planet of learning to assist you on all levels of Knowingness. As we have previously stated, sometimes the journey may seem treacherous, but have faith, Children of Light, and trust that each step on your path is lit with divine glory at this time. It is through surrender and release that you allow the great cosmic flame to stream through your consciousness and ignite the necessary memories to activate within. The keys have already been installed; however, there are certain points in each soul's evolution when they are given the opportunity to ignite this flame of knowledge with the Sacred Light of Spirit. At this time, those particular souls, many of you reading these pages today, will begin to REMEMBER who you are and what you are here to do. We call you forth and ask you to travel the Path of Light with us. We guide and protect you always.

We Are,
The Beings of Light

I AM a Keeper of the Violet Flame

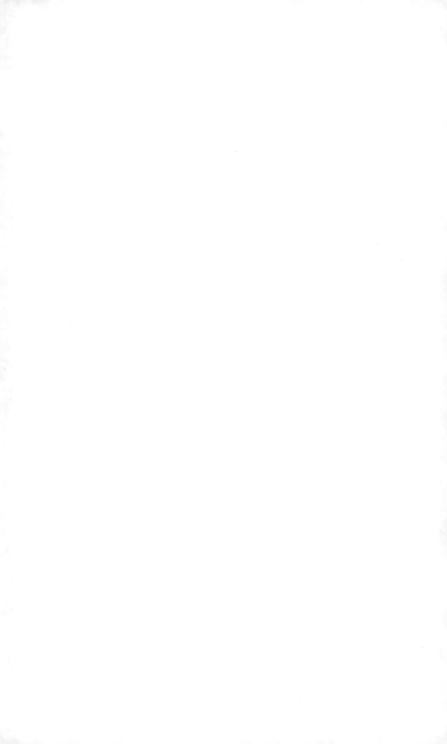

I AM erasing
any negative tendencies now!

Dear Ones . . .
Always remember the importance of
"White Lighting" your vessels.
Each morning, fill every single cell of your bodies with
the pure White Light of Spirit and surround
yourselves with this White Light Protection
and the Golden Light of the Pyramid . . .

I AM surrounding myself
with White Light Protection and
the Golden Light of the Pyramid now!

I AM one with
Infinite Wisdom & Divine Intelligence!

I AM remembering the ancientness of
WHO I AM
and I AM creating my life anew

. . . Does it not feel good, Dear Ones,
to follow the Laws of Spirit and feel confirmation in
your hearts? For when the Laws of Spirit are honored,
your life takes on a whole new ambiance,
filled with the beauty and recognition of the power of
thought, word, and deed, and humanity softens its edge
in the coming Age of Light . . .

I AM beautifully aligned
with the Secret Chamber of my Heart

I AM living in my Highest Potential
in each and every moment!

I AM a clear channel of Light

I AM the perfect picture of health.
Every single cell of my body is radiating
in Divine Perfection!

. . . To ignite the Christ Consciousness within is to take responsibility for your role as a co-creator with Spirit. To carry this torch of light is one of the highest honors of the Heavens, and replenishes your spiritual treasure box . . .

I AM consciously
igniting & living my Christ Light within!

I AM co-creating with Spirit now!

I Love myself, I Know myself, I Trust myself,
I BELIEVE in myself!

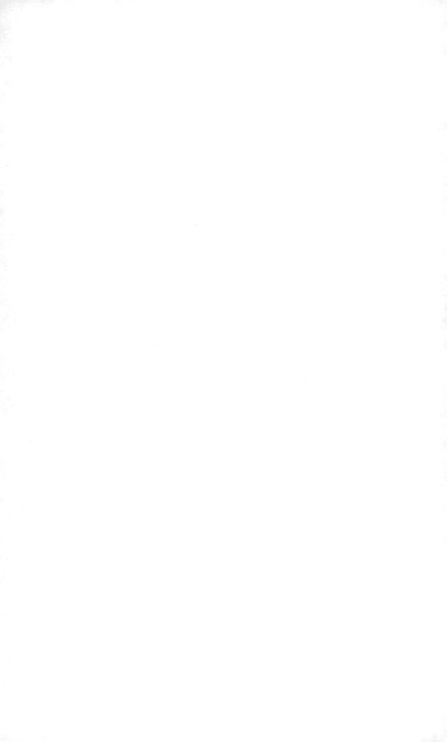

. . . As our planet moves closer to co-creating with Spirit and becoming the glorious, long awaited Heaven on Earth, it is imperative for its inhabitants to raise their vibrational stature to a level that is sufficient enough to integrate and assimilate the amplified frequencies of this new Golden Age of Energy. . .

I AM upgrading my energy system now!

I AM consciously
integrating, assimilating, and sustaining
these high vibrational frequencies!

I AM graciously receiving
gifts from the Universe now!

Greetings Children of Light,

*It matters not what your religion of choice is Dear Ones, for when the Trinity of the **Great Creator** is formed with the **Intention** and **Good of All**, the spark of divinity is ignited in the hearts of all mankind. Be kind and gracious to one other, all around the world, for where there is forgiveness, there is calm. Where there is peace, there is love, and where there is tolerance allowing all people to be who they are, there is UNITY. The Seventh Golden Age is upon us quickly, and we must embrace ALL of our brothers and sisters, and work together in this coming time for our beautiful Planet Earth to make its alignment in the galaxies and transcend into its magnificent, illuminating star. We ask you to embrace the light and assist us with this most vital transition.*

Be guided by Spirit in each moment and the people around you will begin to follow. The time has come for the Allegiance of Light to assemble and soar into action at the very heart of your Being.

We are with you and shall guide and assist you in all of your endeavors.

We Are,
The Beings of Light

I AM love

I AM light

I AM wholeness

I AM clarity

I AM inner truth

I AM peace

I AM compassion

I AM forgiveness

. . . Be full of Gratitude, Dear Ones,
for when you are grateful,
you attract all that is good to you, and you share
in the bounties of Spirit. . .

I AM full of gratitude
in each and every moment!

(acknowledge everything you are grateful for)

Thank you. Thank you. Thank you

I AM embracing life with
freedom, joy & laughter now!

~ If seeking Divine Partnership ~

I AM attracting my spiritual life mate now!

I AM co-creating
magically
with my divine partner now!

I AM creating harmonious relationships
in every area of my life now!

I AM overflowing with Infinite Love,
Grace & Kindness now!

Dear Ones,

Subatomic molecular structure is one that is based on particles or atoms combined with love & compassion of the human energy field. This combination is necessary to creation, to perfect the Adam Kadmon, the ultimate Spiritual Light Being on the earth plane in this new dimensional frequency. For those who wish not to make these preparations and ascend in the Age of Light, they will simply fade from the view of those who are so diligently preparing for the catalystic surge forward. It will be nothing "dramatic" as you say, but heartfelt at the deepest level of your Being. These earthlings will simply be operating at a lesser frequency ~ only one outside of our dimensional range of motion, so to speak. Some of you are worried about certain loved ones or family members making this beautiful shift of alignment into the new Age of Light, but "fear not", as your Great Teacher Sananda has said, for their Ascension will be just as their soul has planned and their mission is in divine order for their maturation on the spiritual plane.

We would like to add here that many of you Spiritual Light Workers have made the necessary spiritual contracts to awaken heartfelt souls and family members closer to the Eve of the Great Ascension; so these souls will be directly aligned with your energies to make the grand shift in our much needed Heaven on Earth, which we have so diligently been in preparation for and have co-created with the Great Source of All. Be in love, Dear Ones, and know that the Divine Gathering of the Ancients surround you and guide you in all of your endeavors.

We await you at the Table of Plenty.

We Are,
The Beings of Light

I AM recoding, reconnecting & reactivating
my 12-strand DNA now!

I AM releasing & clearing
any negative karmic debt from all levels
of my Beingness and my cellular memory
forevermore!

I AM one with Divine Calmness

I AM allowing my inner child to PLAY
and to be heard!

Dear Ones,

We greet you this day with great exuberance and excitement, for you have answered the call within your hearts to step forward and join the Legions of Light to not only transform your own lives, but to assist humanity's Spiritual Evolution, for when you transform yourselves, you assist others in cleansing and purifying the multifaceted Jewel of the Heart. We embrace you and shower you with many gifts of Spirit in the days to come.

We hold a light in our hearts for you, for as you have ignited your own Christ Light within, you begin to soar beautifully into the future, assisting others in their awakening process.

We Are,
The Beings of Light

I AM in perfect alignment with my Higher Self
in service to others

I AM utilizing my Spiritual Gifts
to assist humanity's healing & raise
Conscious Awareness universally!

I AM attracting now
those people that can benefit most from
my work & my energy!

I AM receiving tremendous prosperity
in my life now
for the highest good of all!

I AM guided by my inner Spirit
in each & every moment

I AM inviting blessings into my life now!

Those of you who have answered this call
are the new "Beacons of Light" in the coming age,
assisting humanity in its multidimensional shift
into the Golden Age of Light,
as your planet embraces its long-awaited Ascension.

I AM Being, I AM Knowing,
I AM Allowing, I AM Receiving

. . . We are each blessed with
Angels and beautiful Cosmic Guides.
They await your invitation to blissfully step in and guide
you in all of your endeavors.

Greetings Dear Ones,

As the beautiful lotus bud has opened and awakened to the Light of Spirit, your multifaceted hearts have activated the memory patterns of light deep within your souls. As you embrace the truth and divinity of who you are, your beautiful reflection radiates and illuminates your Christ Light to others and awakens the three-fold flame within the Secret Chamber of their hearts so that they, too, may live in the Light of Spirit.

This multidimensional crystalline structure houses many codes and keys to the awakening soul, each intricate cut and pattern built with the knowledge of each personal soul's awakening to the destiny of Spirit. As the lotus flower trusts and opens its beautiful tender petals, revealing the precious, multifaceted Jewel of the Heart, a matrix is activated, radiating and expanding light across all time and space, healing and transmuting yourselves and the planet.

Blessings and gratitude, Dear Ones, as you have opened the doorways of your Bejeweled Hearts.

We Are,
The Beings of Light

I AM living in my Highest Consciousness now!

I AM creating miracles in my life now!

I AM joyously participating in
healing & nurturing Mother Earth!

I AM radiating LOVE to the World.
The World is at PEACE and in perfect harmony now!

I AM Grateful for ALL that I AM

I AM THAT I AM

THE TIME IS NOW!

Remember these words, Dear Ones,

. . . for they are the Glory of God manifesting in you as you fully soar on your journey of self-discovery and co-creation with Spirit.

We Are,
The Beings of Light

The "Beings of Light"
serve you as part of the team of
The Great White Brotherhood*
beside the Celestial & Spiritual Hierarchy.
Their role and duty to the earth plane is to assist
humanity's healing and raise Conscious Awareness
for the Awakening of Earthlings and, most recently,
for the preparation of the Great Shift
which has already begun on Planet Earth.
They can be called upon at any time for assistance.
The "Beings of Light" are in full gratitude to those
holding these pages and look forward to the
coming Age of Light where we enter peace on earth
in perfect harmony and love for ALL.

*White referring to "LIGHT"